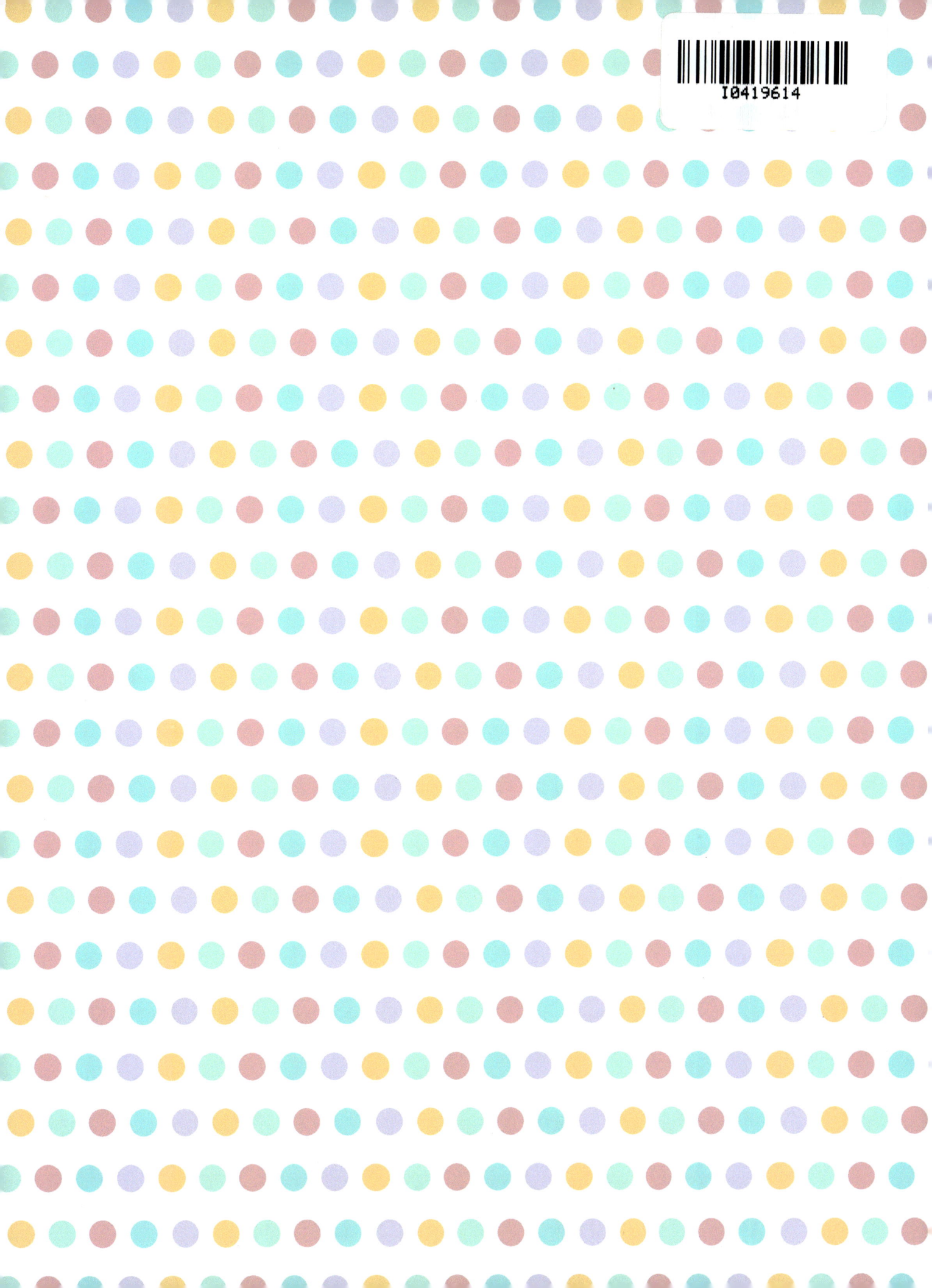

# How to use your new book!

This is **YOUR** book just for you!

Each page has space for you to write a list of special things.

Each list also has some suggestions.

If you like the suggestions, you can highlight them or draw happy faces or mark them with stickers.

If you don't like them, you can cross them out.

Use your stickers and crayons to make this book special.

If you like, you can show it to your daddy or keep it just for you!

# Super shoppy treats wishlist!

Sparkly lip gloss

Puffy stickers

New Coloring Book and crayons

PINK PACI

Super yummy BAth bubbles

New stuffie (must be cute!)

Bows! Pretty hair bows!

_____

_____

_____

_____

_____

_____

_____

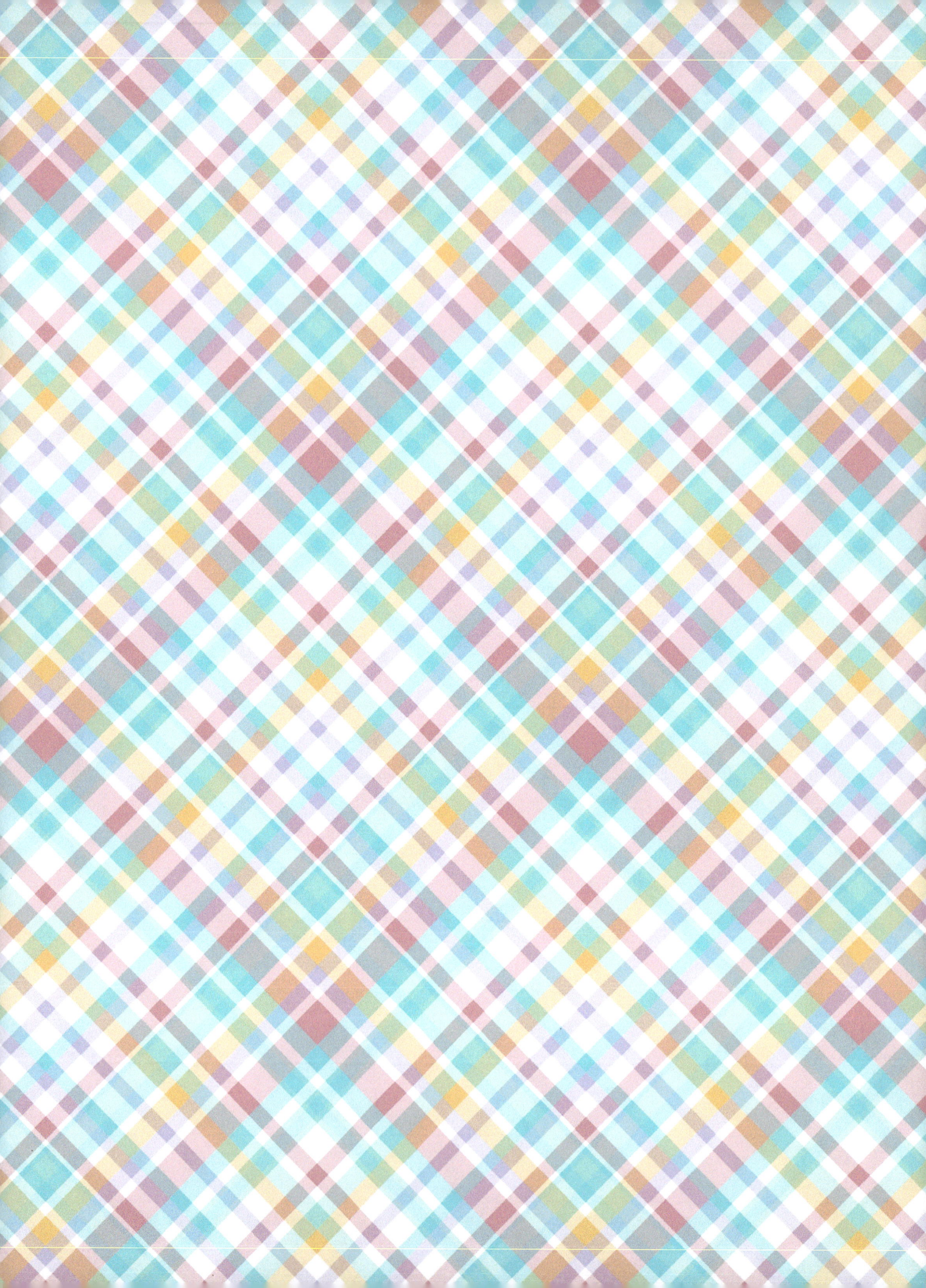

# Things Daddy does for me

Buckles my seatbelt

makes me teeny sandwiches

fills my sippy cup

Buys me candy

Puts my fuzzy sockies on my feet

Holds my hand when we cross the street

_____

_____

_____

_____

_____

_____

_____

## At snuggle time I like

Bedtime stories

Kisses and more kisses

Snugglywuggly pajamas

My favorite blankie

Stuffie cuddles

warm milk

Sucking my paci

_____

_____

_____

_____

_____

_____

_____

_____

# My favorite trips with Daddy

Going to the zoo

Seeing fishies at the aquarium

Princess movies with a **BIG** bucket of popcorn

Ice cream sundaes with every topping!

Feeding duckies at the pond

Swinging on the swings at the park

_____

_____

_____

_____

_____

_____

_____

# Naughty things to do (hee!)

Blow bubbles in my milk

boop daddy on the nose

bite daddy (gently) and run away!

Say, "Missed me, now you hafta kiss me!"

Make prank calls to Daddy (and try not to giggle!)

Spill ice cream on Daddy

_____

_____

_____

_____

_____

_____

_____

# Boo. When I'm naughty...

Spankings
Standing in the corner
Writing lines (boo!)
Going to bed early
Naughty mark on my star chart
Sitting on the naughty step
Broccoli for dinner (ew!)

_____

_____

_____

_____

_____

_____

_____

# Things I call Daddy (uh oh)

Meanieface
Butthead
Poopyface
Sillynose
Stinkyfeet

_____

_____

_____

_____

_____

_____

_____

## Fun things I do on my own!

Play dress up

Pretend to be a kitty or a puppy

Cuddle with an actual kitty or puppy

Bake cuppycakes

solve a **SUPER DIFFICULT** puzzle (100 pieces!)

Blow bubbles in the air

_____

_____

_____

_____

_____

_____

_____

## Secrets I tell my stuffie

I know daddy loves me lots!

I'm scared of the dark (And monsters!)

I'm sleeeepy... but don't tell daddy!

where my secret candy is

_____

_____

_____

_____

_____

_____

_____

# My favorite snackies

Warm milk and cookies

Juice boxes

Goldfish

Teeny cookies

Ice pops

Applesauce

Not broccoli

_____

_____

_____

_____

_____

_____

_____

# My bestest clothes

FLOOFY PARTY DRESS

COSY ROMPER

DINOSAUR OUTFIT

FUZZY SOCKIES

FRILLY NIGHTIE

POLKA DOT SWIMMIES

SNUGGLY ONESIE

_____

_____

_____

_____

_____

_____

_____

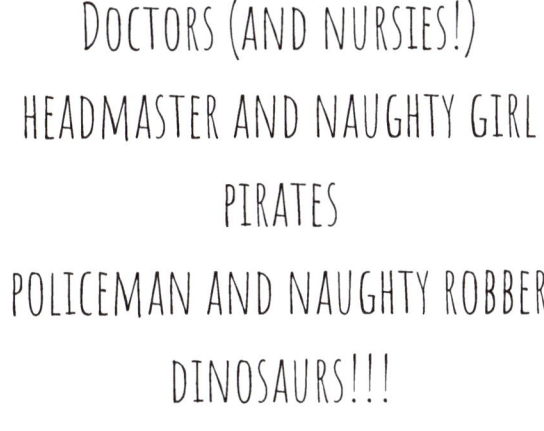

Doctors (and nursies!)

HEADMASTER AND NAUGHTY GIRL

PIRATES

POLICEMAN AND NAUGHTY ROBBER

DINOSAURS!!!

_____

_____

_____

_____

_____

_____

_____

# Ways to make daddy happy

MAKE YUMMY BREAKFAST

FIND HIS GLASSES, TIE OR SHOES

POUR HIM COFFEE (VERY CAREFULLY!  IT'S HOT!)

RUN HIM A BUBBLY BATH WITH LOTS OF BUBBLES

WRITE A STORY FOR HIM AND READ IT

DRAW HIM A PICTURE OF US TOGETHER WITH LOTS OF HEARTS

_____

_____

_____

_____

_____

_____

_____

_____

# Quiet time treats

write a story with Sparkly gel pens

painting my toenails

build a pillow fort and fall asleep in it

read a comic book

make a scrapbook with pictures of friends and kitties

learn to make a cross stitch (watch the pokey needle! Ow!)

_____

_____

_____

_____

_____

_____

_____

## Favorite stuffies

BUNNY

PANDA

LLAMA

TEDDY BEAR

SOFT DOLLY

_____

_____

_____

_____

_____

_____

_____

# Chores I help with

Tidy my room

Fold Daddy's clothes

Make the bed (tidy corners!)

Dust Daddy's desk and organize his things nicely

putting away toys and sparklies

sort books neatly

_____

_____

_____

_____

_____

_____

_____

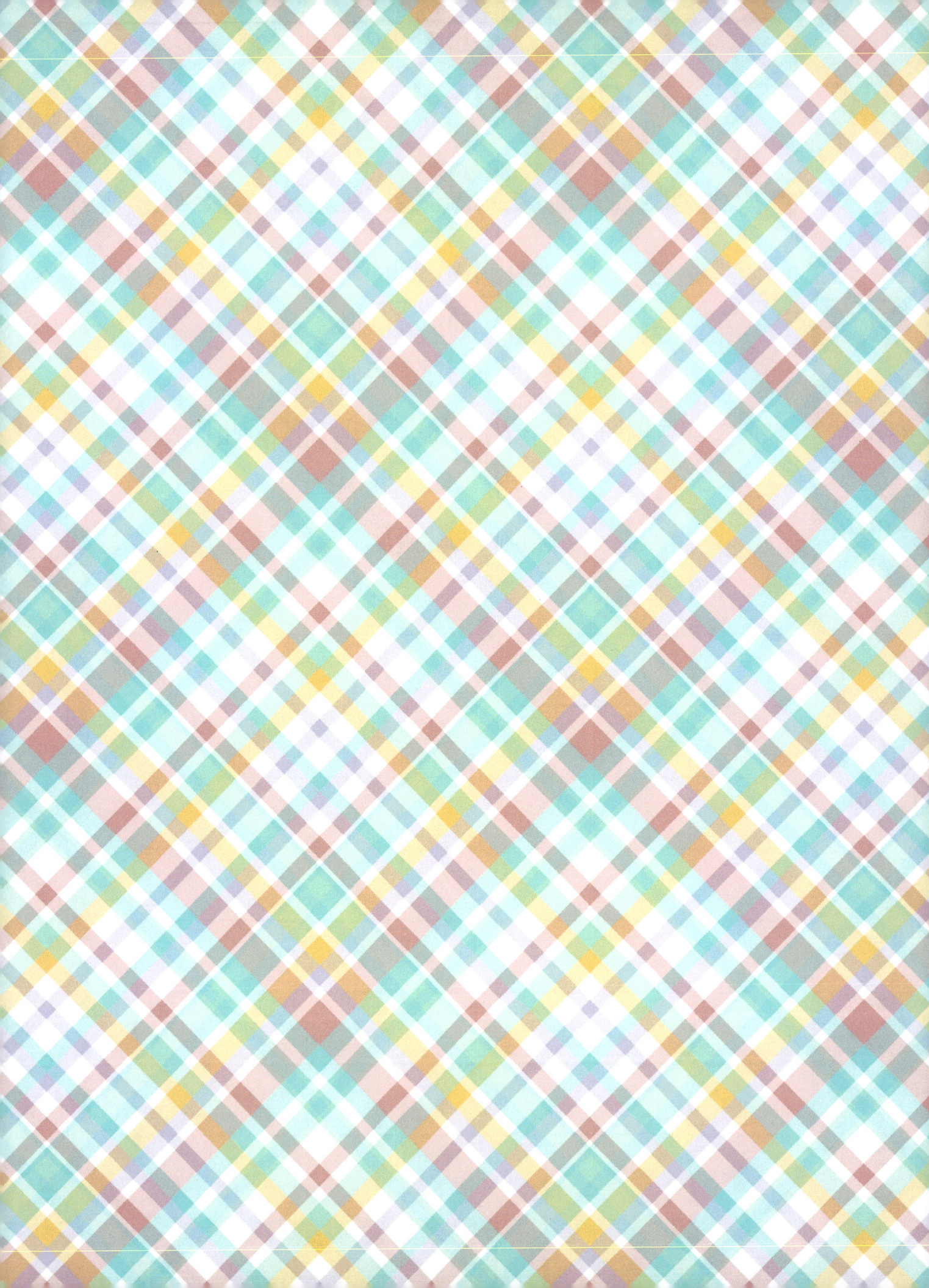

## I make pretty things!

Beading bracelets

sew scrunchies for my hair

Decorate my pacifier

Paint a picture (of Daddy)

make finger puppets for a show

Use stamps to make a picture and color it

_____

_____

_____

_____

_____

_____

_____

# Draw a 'Daddy and Me' picture

## Write a thank you letter

Dear Daddy,

_____

_____

_____

_____

_____

_____

_____

_____

_____

_____

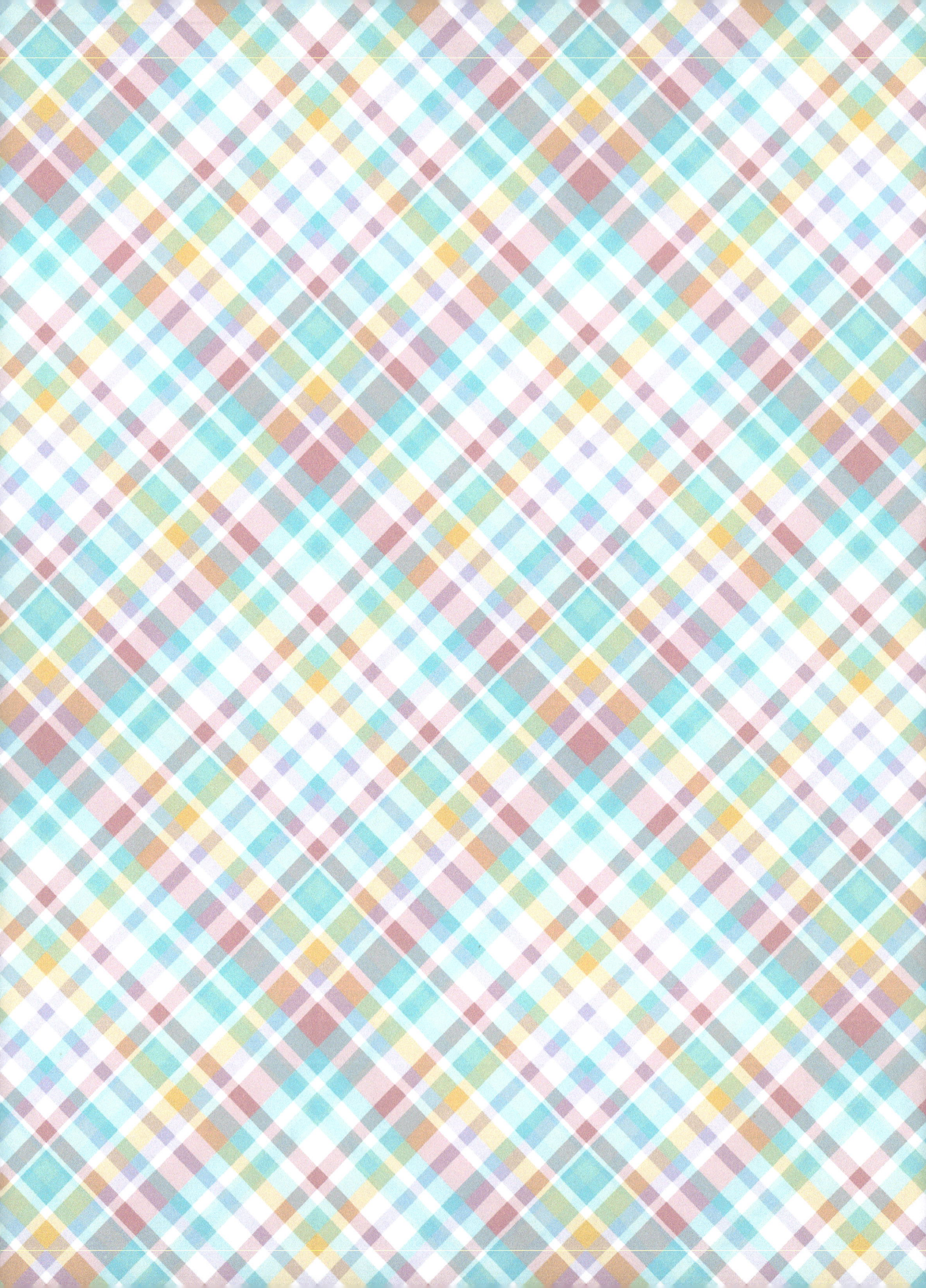

# Responsibility sticker chart

|  | Did my chores | Took care of myself | Took care of Daddy |
|---|---|---|---|
| Monday |  |  |  |
| Tuesday |  |  |  |
| Wednesday |  |  |  |
| Thursday |  |  |  |
| Friday |  |  |  |
| Saturday |  |  |  |
| Sunday |  |  |  |

# Responsibility sticker chart

| | Did my chores | Took care of myself | Took care of Daddy |
|---|---|---|---|
| Monday | | | |
| Tuesday | | | |
| Wednesday | | | |
| Thursday | | | |
| Friday | | | |
| Saturday | | | |
| Sunday | | | |

# Responsibility sticker chart

| | Did my chores | Took care of myself | Took care of Daddy |
|---|---|---|---|
| Monday | | | |
| Tuesday | | | |
| Wednesday | | | |
| Thursday | | | |
| Friday | | | |
| Saturday | | | |
| Sunday | | | |

# Responsibility sticker chart

|  | Did my chores | Took care of myself | Took care of Daddy |
|---|---|---|---|
| Monday |  |  |  |
| Tuesday |  |  |  |
| Wednesday |  |  |  |
| Thursday |  |  |  |
| Friday |  |  |  |
| Saturday |  |  |  |
| Sunday |  |  |  |